A Family Guide to Mental Health Recovery

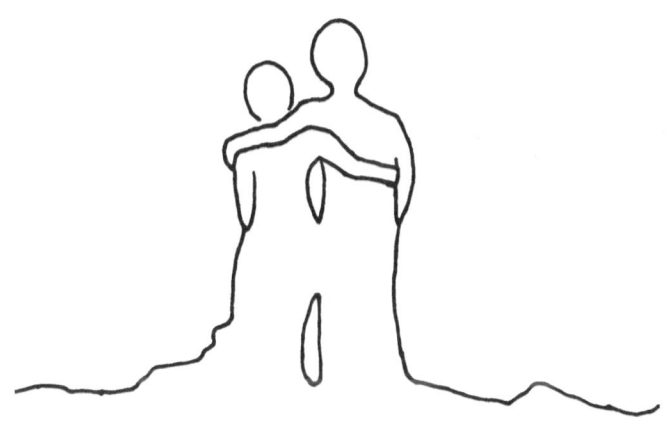

What You Need to Know from Day One

By Virgil Stucker and Stephanie McMahon

ISBN-13: 9798645061722

Thanks to Darcy Whitten of Darcy Whitten Designs for the beautiful drawings; to David Edge of David Edge Design for the great cover design and chapter divider pages; and to Sue Reynard for the editing and layout.

We invite readers to send us their reactions and suggestions for future improvements to: Virgil@VirgilStuckerandAssociates.com

Dedication

This book is dedicated to my wife Elisabeth (Otter) Stucker
who has been my partner and soulmate for nearly 44 years.
As a family, we have lived with, walked with, dined with, and
worked with hundreds of individuals with mental illness. What
a wonderful life it is to share our hearts and minds with some
of the most vulnerable in society and see them survive and
thrive.

Virgil Stucker, April 2020

Preface and Acknowledgments

Let's get personal right up front. This is a difficult time; for some it is a completely overwhelming experience as we try to cope with the health and economic impacts of COVID-19 on the world, on our country and community, and on our family. You are likely reading these words because you are also coping with the mental illness of a family member on top of it all. More than ever you are being called on to help your family member journey through this time of uncertainty toward sustainable recovery from mental illness. My hope is that our guide will help you to become and remain the resilient champion and caregiver that is needed now, more than ever, for your family member.

Who am I to offer guidance to you? At the moment, my wife Lis and I (at 68 and 67) are "hunkered down" and socially distancing in order to remain healthy. Over the Internet and phone, I am continuing to offer consultation to families and mental health leaders, who are under tremendous stress. Looking back, here is a story of some of the experiences in my life that have led me to this moment of wanting to offer a guide to you. It is not a perfect guide, because there are no perfect answers in mental health care. However, if you dig deeply into what we have written, we think you will learn how to help your family member journey successfully toward mental health recovery. Start from day one with a "recovery attitude"; don't give in to experts with perfect answers and don't accept mental illness as a chronic disability.

My story: My high school dream of becoming an astronaut was shattered when I learned in the spring of 1970 of the suicide of a friend in Vietnam. Instead of accepting my appointment to the US Air Force Academy, I pivoted toward 'inner-space' and studied philosophy in college. I tried to apply critical, rational thinking to life's mysteries. I also learned about human vulnerability when I was a math tutor for an autistic boy. He had been freed by authorities from his locked room in his family's house, where the effects of stigma had imprisoned him. As a volunteer probation officer for a disturbed adolescent, I saw again how damaging the world can be to the weakest amongst us.

After college, my first mental health job as a hospital psychiatric orderly offered moments of pain and perplexity. Helping tie a young psychotic man into four-point restraints was jarring. I retreated to the hospital chapel and cried. I was also the designated guide for patients coming to consciousness after electro-convulsive shock treatments, I would say, "Your name is George and this is November 15th..." ECT is indeed a perplexing mental health treatment, but I observed deeply depressed people whose moods immediately improved.

My next stop was to work at Gould Farm, America's oldest therapeutic community for individuals with mental illness. I experienced a new way of serving some of society's most vulnerable members with compassion and hope. My heart and head aligned with Gould Farm's methods for helping individuals, called Guests, feel a renewed sense of belonging and purpose along with strengthened resilience.

This defining time at Gould, which was intended to last for 3 months, turned into many years. I met my wife Lis there and our children Dominic, Christoph, Heidi and Stephanie were born as we shared our lives with 40 mentally ill adults, who resided with us on the Farm's 600-acre, village-like campus. My parents Robert and Florence also worked at Gould Farm for a few years. Lis and I felt called to help start places like Gould Farm.

All the therapeutic communities I helped to start were inspired and fueled by the philanthropy and volunteerism of empowered parents taking action. The first was Gateway Homes in Virginia, which was led by Carol and William Moore. Then,

Rose Hill Center in Michigan, which is still led by Rosemary and Dan Kelly, and then, CooperRiis in North Carolina which is inspired and led by Lisbeth Riis and Don Cooper. Each of these non-profit organizations is a testament to what empowered parents can do to help not only a family member in need, but others as well.

My experiences in these therapeutic communities brought me great joy, but there was also pain. Following my observation of the tragic suicide of a resident in one of these communities that I led, I was overwhelmed by PTSD. EMDR treatment over 9 months helped greatly. I also remember each word and feeling that I had when - more than once - I had to call parents to tell them that their loved one had been overwhelmed by their mental illness and had ended their life. This kind of loss is a deeply unfortunate reality of working and living with people struggling with serious mental illness and it never gets easier to bear for those delivering the care

Over the decades. I have walked with a few thousand families and individuals on their journeys to mental health recovery. I have observed amazing displays of courage, commitment and success. I wish I could name them, but my respect for their privacy holds me back. They know who they are and they know I admire them.

In order to extend my life's joy and meaning, I launched a therapeutic consulting practice with the help of our youngest daughter, Stephanie McMahon, in July 2017. I am deeply grateful that she is the co-author of this guide. She is also a functional medicine health coach and produces a podcast called *Mental Horizons* that hosts discussions with mental health leaders and people with lived experience of mental illness. I have so many reasons for hope and have met many good people on my life's journey.

Virgil Stucker

April 7, 2020

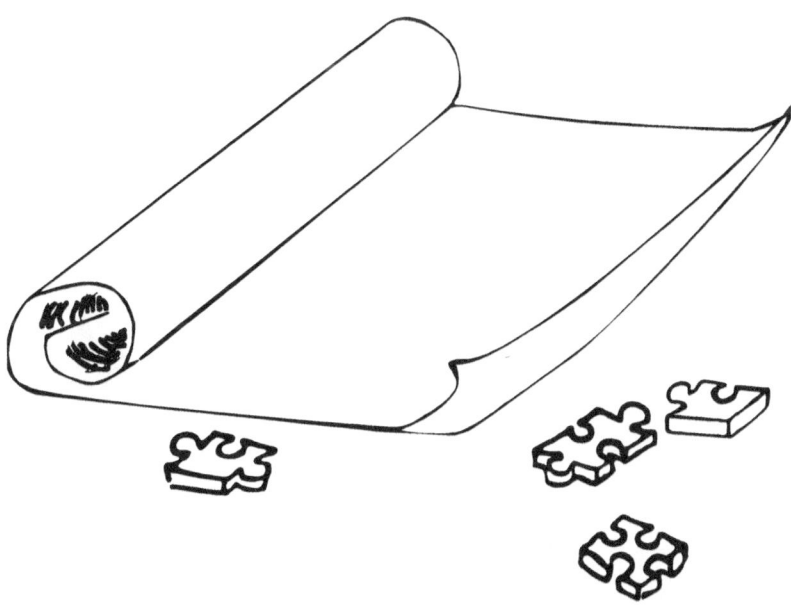

Contents

Prologue

By Virgil Stucker

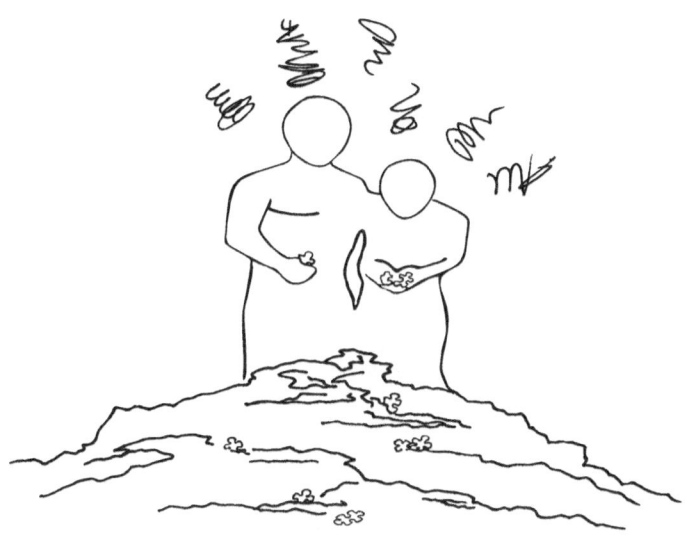

Where are you on the journey through the mental health system?

Perhaps your family member or friend has entered the hospital for the first time and you feel desperate...

Perhaps your family member has had multiple hospitalizations and you feel bewildered...

Perhaps your family member is doing fairly well but needs on-going care and support, and you feel exhausted and terrified about what will happen to them when you are not around...

In all cases, we think this guide will help you plot a path to answers that may work for you and your family member.

Over the decades I have been invited into hundreds of conversations with families whose lives have been disrupted by mental illness. Although each story is unique, these families are often equally overwhelmed, anxious, exhausted, fearful, and confused. Each family has realized there is no perfect solution but has not given up. In listening closely, I generally discover and try to build on their remaining hope, curiosity, and will to survive as a family.

We are coming out of a dark time for mental health care, which some called a crisis even before COVID-19 disrupted our lives. At the moment, some programs and even some psychiatric units and ER's have discharged their patients or clients, sending them to unprepared homes or to homeless shelters. Overnight, tele-health services have become the norm. At the same time, many courageous mental health leaders have persevered, continuing to operate their care and treatment programs under severely constrained circumstances. Many of the best are non profit programs operating with new financial strains because the resources of their donors have been diminished.

As we move beyond the COVID-19 crisis, we believe we will be a kinder and gentler society with renewed energy to help the vulnerable amongst us. At this point, however, we are uncertain what the "new normal" will be for the mental health care world. Some current services will not survive; some will merge. Tele-health services will likely expand. Some will create new services to help families re-assemble their understanding of available services and navigate their journey to gain access to them.

Even before COVID-19, here are some of the challenges faced by families in their quest to become 'resilient champions' for their loved ones.

After the mid-1900s when the courts, pressured by public opinion, closed most mental hospitals and institutions, often with over a thousand 'beds' each, we went too far. In 1950, the US had 550,000 psychiatric hospital beds; by 2016, the number had dropped to 37,679.[1] The promised community-based services that were intended under President Kennedy's administration 50 years ago never fully materialized. The remaining system is now fractured into disconnected pieces.

Over 392,000 individuals with serious mental illness reside in jail or prison and over 110,000 are homeless on the streets. Many reside in the homes of aging parents who are anxious about what will happen to their family members after they can no longer care for them. As of 2016, about 8.4 million families

---

1   The numbers reported on this page were included in a Washington Post Op Ed by Joe Grogan, director of the Domestic Policy Council on February 9, 2020.

were caring for a family member with mental illness whose average age was 45.[2]

Record numbers of students entering college already have a diagnosed mental illness; some may be well treated and be prepared to be successful students... but the stress is greater than they have ever experienced. The sophomore year seems to be the most stressful. This is the year when students who have not been previously diagnosed may also suddenly appear to have a mental health breakdown. The student may turn for help to a college mental health counselor who often already has an overwhelming caseload of a few hundred students.

We hope for a better future for these individuals. Indeed, imagine a future where the quest for recovery starts earlier and results less frequently in the individual losing hope and becoming chronically mentally ill. This future is still attainable.

Unfortunately, the national dialogue has been more about fear than compassion. Stigma spawns silence. People with a mental illness often have a hard time engaging with their environment. When someone loses their sense of social belonging, they can quickly become isolated. And isolation often leads to declines in both physical and mental health.

---

2   https://www.caregiving.org/circleofcare/

Humans are social creatures and we tend to thrive when we feel a sense of greater purpose, connection, and belonging. We get uncomfortable when someone behaves in ways that go against accepted behaviors.

How can families courageously find a way through this deafening silence and help their family members? There are ways!

There are existing pieces of the mental health care system that, with good planning, can be woven into a continuum of treatment options for these individuals. Without this planning, however, mental health treatment consists too often only of a high-pressure, short-term hospital stay followed by an occasional outpatient clinical appointment. In between is a void when what individuals need is a mix of services.

> If you feel desperate or are experiencing an emergency, call 911. Otherwise, "break the glass" and read and perhaps re-read the material in this guide. It may feel initially a bit intense or dense, but we think that it will add value to your journey.

The recovery process can be long and arduous. We respect, too, that sometimes, no matter what a family caregiver has done or may do, their loved one simply may not be able to progress beyond their need for care and permanent support. In this situation, a goal of "maintenance" rather than "progress" may be a worthy choice. After all, the process and outcomes are highly individualized.

We want this guide to inspire, inform and activate families who are just beginning the recovery journey with their loved one as well as at any point along the journey. We want to help you—at all stages of recovery—to be a champion and an empowered caregiver for your loved one. This guide will urge you to move even more courageously into being a full member on the team of experts who will be treating and caring for your family member. In fact, we will urge your family member to be on the recovery team as well, right in the middle of it.

Too frequently, as a championing family member you are asked to step aside, even though you may be fully expert in your family member's needs. (Yes, you may also be a part of the problem, but you can also always be a part of the solution.) Too frequently, the rush to diagnostic judgment in the early chaos of a mental health crisis is shown later to have led to inaccurate, short-sighted conclusions. Too often, the person with mental illness is defined as a 'patient' and separated from their loved ones with no champion fighting with them for their recovery. Too often these individuals succumb to a system that focuses more on treating their symptoms than on encouraging them still to dream and strive for a functional and fulfilled life. As a result they may end up in a diminished state of chronic disability and need a perpetual caregiver more than they need a champion.

This guide calls forth champions, humble but resilient champions and caregivers, to arise. "Humble"? Yes, because the reader will see there are no perfect answers. But don't give up. Resiliency is called for! Also the best answers are individualized and achieved over time when a courageous family member or friend is joined by the person with mental illness who also becomes a champion of their own recovery. Together, you can seek clear understandings of diagnoses and best treatments while helping your family member to pursue the dream of achieving a life of belonging, purpose and resilience.

There will be a better day and we hope that this guide will help you and your family member to reach that day.

You can find stories like these and other solution-oriented interviews with and writings from mental health leaders referenced on our blog and podcast, all housed on our website, VirgilStuckerandAssociates.com.

Improving Care For Your Loved One

The stories about mental illness can be heart wrenching. Most families have had moments of fearing the worst. Some have experienced it. The days and nights can be filled with anxiety and one's will to be well can be worn down. Even the mental health care providers may get to the point of saying, "There is nothing more that we can do."

No! We must push forward, keep the dream and hope alive! I have journeyed with people who have come close to falling into the abyss, only to turn their lives around at the last moment. For example, just listen to our Mental Horizons podcast episode with Robert Francis who wrote the book, *On Conquering Schizophrenia*. He is a survivor of schizophrenia and has been a psychotherapist for 12 years. Or listen to our podcast with Elyn Saks who became an attorney and a Ph.D. psychoanalyst despite her schizophrenia. She is also a MacArthur Fellow.

(Note: This is the first time we are using the term 'schizophrenia'. The reader should know that terms like 'psychotic spectrum disorder' are becoming more helpful, since psychotic processes exist across a broad spectrum of symptoms with recommended treatments also being broader than just taking medication.)

Improved care and treatment can motivate your loved one to achieve and sustain a fulfilling and functional life... perhaps not a perfect life, but a good life. Our guide is intended to give you and your family member the hope you will need to successfully plan and navigate the recovery journey.

What's In This Guide

Although this guide is designed to empower the mental health decision making of families dealing with the mental illness of an adult child, it also applies when a sibling is helping a sibling or when an adult child is helping a mentally ill parent or a spouse is helping a spouse. It can also empower friends who may function as champions when families are less involved. When you read "family member" or "loved one", it is meant to apply in each category. This guide may also serve as a resource for the professionals who are on the mental health recovery teams with these resilient champions.

Importantly, this guide also has value for the person who is on his or her own—although the challenges of self-care-giving require even more courage and self-advocacy.

Chapter 1: Understanding Your Situation is designed to help you establish a starting point for moving forward. It describes critical information you need to gather and clarifies the two key questions for you to ask your loved one. The goal is to develop an overall recovery plan that is person-centered, not symptom-centered.

Chapter 2: Becoming a Resilient Champion describes specific steps you can take based on your situation. The recommendations are based on qualitative interviews with families who have cared for a loved one with mental illness. We believe you will find yourself in one or more of these stories. This section will help you feel less alone and become more aware of what it takes to be a resilient champion.

Chapter 3: Understanding Treatment and Care Options is our effort to define current options for mental health care. This chapter aims to help the reader see how these options can fit together to give their family members the care and treatment they need to recover from their mental illness. The recommendations go beyond crisis stabilization, offering a comprehensive, achievable overview of care.

Chapter 4: An Uncertain Path and **Chapter 5: Struggles and Hope** provide a broad overview of the evolution of mental health care over the last 200 years. If you have ever wondered how our mental health system got the way it is today, these chapter sections will help to answer that question. Your increased awareness of the imperfections of mental health care will make you a wiser and more empowered partner of your family member's recovery team.

This booklet is meant to be guidance and is not meant to be individually prescriptive. You will need to rely on the licensed mental health care professionals on your team for their prescriptive knowledge.

Finding Hope and Power

Based on input we received, this guide is for families who are dealing with every stage of their family member's mental illness. We hope that in reading this guide you'll see that there are no *perfect* answers. But there are indeed answers and there is hope for recovery. Your family member can have a fulfilling and functional life despite his or her mental illness.

While the mental health system may be in crisis, we hope that this guide will help you to see and access better care and treatment for your loved one. We hope you do not have to spend one more day feeling powerless.

Chapter 1

Understanding Your Situation

By Virgil Stucker

You may not be able to fully solve your loved one's illness, but you can take action to help them while you also begin to reclaim your own wellbeing. In this chapter, we want you to get off to a good start by gathering information that will be critical in determining the best course of action for your family and your loved one.

Setting a Baseline

Families often feel confused and overwhelmed when they first realize that a loved one may have a mental illness. Before deciding what to do, it's helpful if you gather some basic information in three areas:

1) What the diagnosis is.

2) Which professionals are already involved.

3) What treatment options are already being used or are being considered.

Here is more detail on each of these areas.

A. How sick is my loved one? Are they experiencing more than one sickness?

What do you actually know for a fact about your loved one's diagnosis and current environment?

One issue that will determine how urgent it is that you seek care and what kinds of care is appropriate is known as the "level of acuity." The more dangerous to self or others, the more intense and needy, the more irrational your family member is, the higher is their level of acuity and the greater is their need for intervention and treatment. If the situation is deemed very acute, it will be urgent for your loved one to receive care quickly and perhaps to seek out advanced types of treatment.

You need to ask:

- Are they in a place or situation where they are safe (and will be safe in the near future)?

- Are they dangerous to themselves or others?

- What are their symptoms?

- Is their distress increasing?

You also want to evaluate how complex their situation is. Issues that affect complexity include:

- Which signs of mental illness they are displaying.

- Whether they are abusing substances, illegal drugs or alcohol.

- If they complain about *physical* pain in addition to *emotional* pain.

- If they have a developmental or neurological diagnosis that could cause symptoms of mental illness.

An understanding of both **acuity** and **complexity** will help you decide what level and types of treatment will be most appropriate for your loved one. (We give an overview of the options in Chapter 3.)

B. Who are the professionals already involved?

To get a fuller understanding of the complexity and acuity of your family member's illness, you will need help from mental health professionals. If your family member already sees a professional, nothing prevents you from sharing information you may have about your observations of complexity and acuity. If you don't think the current professionals have a realistic or comprehensive understanding of your family member's condition, you may want to ask where and how you can obtain a more thorough assessment. The professionals involved, however, may be limited in what they can provide to you, depending upon whether your family member allows them to communicate with you.

C. What are the option(s) for care and treatment? Which will work best for my family member?

In addition to figuring out how complex and acute your loved one's situation is, you also have to think through how to tailor any treatment and care to their needs. And you have to consider their willingness to accept either. Chapter 3 describes the range of options in detail.

Here are some examples of the choices you'll face:

- Many people like to talk about what is going on with their thinking and emotions. For them discussing reasons for their distress through psychotherapy may be a cornerstone. There is a range of talk-based therapy treatments available that go by labels such as DBT (dialectical behavior therapy), CBT (cognitive-behavior therapy), EMDR (eye movement desensitization and reprocessing), psychoanalysis and mentalization.

- Many other people prefer to take a more active approach by improving their nutrition and physical fitness, or by meditating. For them, mindfulness, special dietary training and structured physical exercise, work and social/recreational activities may be better initial choices. (Often, several of these approaches are combined. They go by labels such as "integrative psychiatry," "functional medicine," and "nutritional psychiatry.")

- Many people think their distress is best addressed by focusing on their brain's chemical or electro-magnetic processes. For them, psycho-active medications and/or neuroscientific techniques known at TMS (transcranial magnetic stimulation), ECT (electroconvulsive therapy) and neuro-feedback may be cornerstones.

- For people whose mental distress is linked to substance abuse, treatment options that address both issues are often the best choice.

- If they think that their mental and emotional distress is related to a physical or medical condition, they may seek expertise to help them understand and treat their medical and mental health conditions simultaneously.

Think of these options as access paths that your loved one will walk on their journey to recovery. But note that the best outcomes are often achieved when people weave many different approaches into their treatment plan.

Not all professionals are fully aware of the range of options for care and treatment. They and you may—in the moment—be simply focused on stabilizing a crisis. When you get a moment to breathe, do your own research (starting with Chapter 3), keep detailed notes, and suggest options to your family members and to their professional(s). Even hospital discharge planners and private psychiatrists or psychotherapists may lack the information they need. You can help them with your experience, knowledge, and insights.

Developing a Recovery Plan

Once you have a baseline of information, you can work with your loved one on developing a plan for their treatment and care. But "treatment" is just one aspect of creating a path forward—your family member will also benefit from having an individual recovery plan that will help them believe that a better future is possible.

This recovery plan should be a written document with clear goals and objectives that emerge out of the answers to the following questions:

1) **What are your symptoms and what is your diagnosis? (Or diagnoses?)**—This will help you understand how your loved one currently views their situation and the impediments you will face. You and your loved one will have to successfully deal with the impediments posed by the symptoms of diagnosis, freeing the person so that forward movement can occur.

2) **What is your dream?** This question about the dream helps the person chart a path toward their vision of leading a successful life, while they continue working hard to make sure that symptoms are well managed and do not become impediments again.

Too frequently, mental health practitioners who help with treatment planning stop after exploring a patient's diagnosis. It is just as important to discuss the dream question with patients. Thinking about what they want for their future will help motivate your loved one to succeed. They need to believe that they will actually feel better and function better. They need to believe they can reach for their goals for better living. (They also need to feel your belief in their ability to reach their goals.)

Over the years I have asked this dream question of hundreds of people. Sometimes people are puzzled. They'll say things like "I don't know, no one has asked me that question for a long time." As I continue to discuss their dreams with these people, I have sometimes felt like an archaeologist in search of treasure. Most often a glimpse of a dream emerges and, as it does, the person's voice grows stronger.

The discussion of dreams should not be a one-time event. Keep talking to your loved one about what they want for their future. That will help you identify core goals and objectives, and develop specific plans for implementation.

Like "recovery colleges," therapeutic communities (residential treatment centers) may provide services that will help individuals clarify their dreams and develop more awareness that they can actually lead meaningful and purposeful lives. For those who do not need the residential support of therapeutic communities, a coach or mentor may also assist them with dreaming again and striving for a better life. Working on managing one's diagnosis is only half of the recovery journey.

How to get it done

Ideally, the individual with mental illness will work with their loved ones to develop the recovery plan as well as their treatment plan. The recovery plan should:

- Be designed based on an understanding of the person's dreams as well as their diagnosis.

- Document who is on the recovery team and what role each person is playing. This includes which mental health practitioners are doing what, by when and for what result to assist this individual with their recovery

- Be reviewed regularly and updated if needed. The individual and their team can celebrate achievements and discuss what support is needed to see continued progress.

As the recovery plan is implemented, the person will often experience...

- A greater sense of belonging in the world

- A restored capacity for maintaining relationships

- A greater sense of purpose and meaning (related to education, work and fulfillment activities

- Greater independence as they learn how to better manage their illness and achieve their goals

All of this will help the person avoid being thrown off course when symptoms arise again.

Finding Support

If there were only one thing we could change immediately about the reality of mental illness, it would be how the illness isolates people socially from one another. Champions and those experiencing the symptoms of mental illness often struggle to connect with each other and with others because of the stigma they face, the chronic nature of mental illness, and the lack of supportive resources.

That's why we urge you to consider joining a support group. Some groups meet in person. Other groups meet online. You can find these support groups by asking around locally in your

area. Here are some groups found nationally, which you will
need to assess individually.

- Network of Care

- NAMI Family Support Groups

- Al-Anon Support Groups

- DBSA Support Alliance (Depression and Bipolar)

- Mental Health America

- SARDAA (Schizophrenia and Related Disorders Alliance of America)

- ADAA (Anxiety and Depression Association of America)

- OCD Support Groups (International OCD Foundation)

- Family Connections (National Education Alliance for Borderline Personality Disorder)

Taking Action

You and your loved one will face many decisions in the days
to come. Answering the questions and exploring the areas
described in this chapter can help you get off to a good start.
These decisions should be based on what your loved one
wants for their future, not just where they are today.

In the next chapter, we'll continue the emphasis on taking action by describing steps you can take based on the specific concerns you have.

Chapter 2

The Parent Experience

By Stephanie McMahon

Parents supporting adult children with serious mental illness need to have access to professionals willing and able to support the supporter; to act as an arm to lean on in difficult situations. Parents also need a trustworthy and available source of information that will treat them and their loved one as individuals and not numbers in a system.

How can families better support one another in reaching out for help, before a workable situation turns into a full-blown crisis? Awareness of the common stumbling blocks on this path is the first step.

In 2016, co-author Stephanie McMahon along with her classmate Kali Duggins, while completing Master's degrees at Johns Hopkins University, conducted qualitative interviews with parents across the country who had experience supporting an adult child with serious mental illness. In this guide, we've used five themes that emerged from the interviews as a way to discuss common concerns that families have and steps they can take to address those concerns. These themes are:

1) **The emotional and mental health of an adult child is the primary concern**

2) **Mistrust of the mental health system**

3) **Feeling helpless and confused**

4) **Finding professional help is challenging**

5) **Residential treatment viewed as a "worst case" scenario**

You'll find more description of these themes along with relevant quotes from our interviewees and specific actions you can take in each area.

Theme 1: Emotional And Mental Health Of Children Is a Primary Concern

When it comes to the overall wellbeing of their child, the majority of parents who participated in the interviews were most concerned about their emotional and mental health. The people we interviewed said they had been concerned about their child's behavior for some time. Most of them had tried to help their child get treatment for a range of issues such as depression, ADHD, and mood fluctuations.

Here's what the parents told us:

- "I worry if she'll ever be normal and feel good about herself."

- "I worry about keeping them grounded and confident in who they are."

- "Reaching out for help is uncomfortable for a lot of young adults."

- "He was already seeing a psychiatrist" and "Both my boys have seen counselors for several years, and my oldest has been hospitalized after what seemed to be a suicide attempt."

- "Our oldest daughter has always been really down on things. We haven't been sure if she's depressed, but some of the other stuff seems like she is."

Action steps if you are concerned about emotional and mental health

You'll have an easier time talking about mental health issues with your adult child if you start when they are young . Do this even if you don't see specific signs of mental illness. You want "mental health" to be a topic that your family can talk about openly no matter the age of your child:

- Make it a priority to talk with them about mental health and about emotions.

- Learn to acknowledge the challenges your child is going through without trying to fix them. For example, someone may see their child's grades drop in college and instead of reacting by trying to get their grades back up, find out *why* their grades are dropping in the first place. Do not assume you know why the grades have dropped, but instead enter into conversation with your child with curiosity and compassion. If a mental health issue is the root cause of the dropping grades, you will have better luck finding out with this approach.

- Consider the shame surrounding mental illness and the part you play in perpetuating the silence. You are not to blame, but all of us carry a sense of stigma that prevents us from revealing a mental health struggle.

- Lead by example for your loved ones and learn to share your own experience. The more you put words to how this all feels, the easier it becomes to describe.

- Taking care of yourself is an important part of empowering yourself to best help your child. You will be surprised that, once you begin to share openly, others will begin to share too. Do your part to normalize mental illness.

Theme 2: Mistrust of the Mental Health System

The majority of parents who participated in our study reported bad experiences with the mental health system. They said they were often confused or frustrated. The majority have felt like the services they received fell short of their needs and that their loved one was not treated as an individual.

Here are some typical comments from the participants in our study:

- "It was a nightmare. We were treated like baggage and like we were stupid."

- "With my daughter, I've just felt helpless and like people were walking textbooks, spouting off the latest trend."

- "My only understanding is that the system fails more than not."

- "Switched to a different therapist for 1 year, not much improvement. The therapist says 'you are OK.' Maybe another third person will do the trick? Thinking of switching once again."

- "...when our son had a suicide attempt, we did not have a good experience; the doctor just wanted to medicate him. There are aspects of it, when a crisis happens, that need to be improved."

Action steps if you've had negative experiences

You probably already know that dealing with the mental health system can be frustrating. You can't do much to change the system. But you can control how you react to it. And you can get better at dealing with it.

- Become aware of the limitations of the services in your area and understand that the mental health system in every state is overburdened.

- Set realistic expectations so that you are prepared for when the mental health system lets you down.

- Keep detailed records of your loved one's care.

- Know your rights and the resources available to you.

- Thank your providers and partner with them. Most people working in mental health are there because they care about helping people.

Theme 3: Feeling Helpless and Confused

The parents in our interviews were the primary support for their child who had a mental illness. About half also coordinated all the logistics of care: making appointments, making sure the child got to appointments, and so on. They, like the many other people we've talked to, said they often feel confused and unsure of what to do.

The situation is often made worse because mental illness makes it difficult for people to connect with each other, even for those who are parent and child.

Here's a sample of what the parents we interviewed said to us:

- "It's been like I have been trying to hold something together that's bigger than us and we can't really do that very well. Because it's a broken thing and a broken person."

- "I am their caretaker, scheduler, and transportation. I travel with my little calendar everywhere."

- "It wasn't clear for a long time what or if something was really wrong, so we just waited, thinking she'd grow out of it. When she didn't, we thought we couldn't handle it, so we asked her regular doctor to help and set us up with someone if they could."

- "I was more on the periphery. We had a close relationship eventually. But when the illness was unmanaged, it pushed me away. I felt unsafe."

Action Steps If You Feel Helpless and Confused

When it comes to serious mental illness and addiction issues, there is no family member who can do it all.

- Be proactive. Reach out to anyone and everyone involved in helping your child get treatment. Ask questions until you get answers you understand.

- Find support groups—either locally or online—and start sharing your experience. Others have been here before you and you are not alone.

- Recognize that this is a learning process. It takes time to understand the root causes of your child's illness and what treatments are going to work.

- Understand that you are not responsible for solving this problem. In fact, there is no "solution" that will make the problem go away permanently.

- Be kind to yourself and to everyone else involved in this process. Try to maintain your compassion.

Theme 4: Finding Professional Help Is Challenging

The majority of parents interviewed stated that they found lots of information online about care and treatment options, but information about people and groups who could provide support was scarce. They told us they try to exhaust all options before reaching outside their families or support networks for professional help.

When faced with a mental health crisis, all those interviewed stated that they would turn to emergency services then rely on the hospital staff to determine the next steps. The majority of participants stated that their health insurance companies have not been helpful in finding treatment options.

Our interviewees described the challenges this way:

- "I think we have access to options but no support. So I don't know what we really have access to."

- "It was a trial and error process to find the right therapist."

- "We tried looking at reviews but people aren't really so apt to review their therapists!"

- "I think the best thing is to call 911 during a crisis and let them handle everything after that. I would assume that the doctors at the hospital would take care of the rest if they needed to go to a program."

- "We've talked to our regular medical practice and they just gave us a list. They didn't really help."

Action Steps if finding professional help has been challenging

- Recognize that the public mental health system is overburdened and there is a shortage of psychiatrists and therapists. Don't be surprised if you have trouble getting access to facilities or providers even when you know what you want.

- Explore groups such as OpenPath Psychotherapy Collective, who are using technology in creative ways to connect therapists with people in need all over the country. Crisis Text Line is another resource anyone can use; it's free and all it requires is a mobile phone.

- Seek out these creative resources and when you find them, lean on them for guidance.

Theme 5: Residential Treatment Seen As "Worst Case Scenario" Option

Even though only a few families interviewed had had any experience with residential treatment, most considered the concept of 'residential treatment facilities' to have a bad reputation. The majority of people we interviewed were never referred to a residential treatment program by a mental health professional. Mental health professionals had suggested the option in passing to some of our families interviewed, but there was little follow-up.

This lack of direct experience with residential treatment likely contributes to the poor image that many people have of it. The people we interviewed described hospital-like or locked-room settings when imagining a residential setting,

The same inexperience may also explain why the majority of people we interviewed thought residential treatment was needed only when someone might pose a harm to themselves or others. Others saw residential treatment as a last resort, needed only when all other options have been exhausted. Neither group ever felt things were "bad enough" to warrant residential treatment for their children or loved ones.

To describe it in their own words:

- "Never thought it was to the point that I needed that much help. If I felt that they needed it, I would not think twice. I would reach out. As a pride thing, I feel like that would be my last resort."

- "I know about 12-Step and rehab, but for depression and stuff, I only think of padded walls and drugs. It's always seemed sad to me. I don't know much about them."

- "Residential treatment sounds scary. Do you live at a hospital?"

- "[Hospital staff] told us that a residential program was what was needed, but no one helped us find one. The team at the hospital sent us away like he was cured and told us to follow up with a counselor and maybe think about some meds."

Action Steps If You're Concerned About Residential Treatment

- Residential treatment is not for everyone. If you have a strong support network of family and friends and professional support and are able to work and maintain relationships, then going to residential treatment may not be for you. But if your mental health or substance abuse issues have gotten in the way of your relationships and disrupted your education and career activities, then residential treatment may be a fit; in fact, it may be the thing that makes all the difference.

- If you listen to families who did finally seek out residential treatment, you hear them wish they had sought it out sooner. Instead of spending a lot of time and money on one outpatient remedy or therapy after another, they wish they had considered the comprehensive care offered by residential treatment programs sooner, before it was a last resort.

- If this feels like you, we encourage you to challenge the stereotypes about residential treatment you might hold in your mind. Learn about the good programs out there; call them and visit them to see for yourself. The good ones will welcome you in, explain their programs fully, and give you a tour. Most families are surprised to see that these can be incredibly healing, supportive spaces and not at all what they feared.

Empowering Yourself

With all the challenges they face, it's easy for families to feel confused and helpless when dealing with mental illness. This chapter is focused on helping you move forward by describing specific actions linked to the five major concerns that families have. We hope this will get you started down a path where you feel more empowered to cope with your situation.

Action Summary Table

Concern	Action
The emotional and mental health of an adult child is the primary concern	• Make it a priority to talk with them about mental health and about emotions. • Learn how to acknowledge the challenges your child is going through without trying to fix them. • Consider the shame surrounding mental illness and the part you play in perpetuating the silence. You are not to blame, but all of us carry a sense of stigma that prevent us from revealing a mental health struggle. • Lead by example for your loved ones and learn to share your own experience. The more you put words to how this all feels, the easier it becomes to describe. • Taking care of yourself is an important part of empowering yourself to best help your child. You will be surprised that, once you begin to share openly, others will begin to share too. Do your part to normalize mental illness.

Concern	Action
Mistrust of the mental health system	• Become aware of the limitations of the services in your area and understand that the mental health system in every state is overburdened.
	• Set realistic expectations so that you are prepared for when the mental health system lets you down.
	• Keep detailed records of your loved one's care.
	• Know your rights and the resources available to you.
	• Thank your providers and partner with them. Most people working in mental health are there because they care about helping people

Concern	Action
Feeling helpless and confused	• Be proactive. Reach out to anyone and everyone involved in helping your child (or other family member) get treatment. Ask questions until you get answers you understand.
	• Find support groups—either locally or online—and start sharing your experience. Others have been here before you and you are not alone. See p. 33 for advice on finding a group near you.
	• Recognize that this is a learning process. It takes time to understand the root causes of your family member's illness and what treatments are going to work.
	• Understand that you are not responsible for solving this problem. In fact, there is no "solution" that will make the problem go away permanently.
	• Be kind to yourself and to everyone else involved in this process. Try to maintain your compassion

Concern	Action
Finding professional help is challenging	• Recognize that the public mental health system is overburdened and there is a shortage of psychiatrists and therapists. Don't be surprised if you have trouble getting access to facilities or providers even when you know what you want. • Explore groups such as OpenPath Psychotherapy Collective, who are using technology in creative ways to connect therapists with people in need all over the country. Crisis Text Line is another resource anyone can use; it's free and all it requires is a mobile phone. • Seek out these creative resources and when you find them, lean on them for guidance
Residential treatment viewed as a "worst case" scenario	• Residential treatment is not for everyone. But if your mental health issues have gotten in the way of your relationships and disrupted your education and career activities, then residential treatment may be a fit; in fact, it may be the thing that makes all the difference. • If you listen to families who finally seek out residential treatment, you hear them wish they had sought it out sooner. • We encourage you to challenge the stereotypes about residential treatment you might hold in your mind. Learn about the good programs out there: call them and visit them to see for yourself.

Chapter 3

Bridging the Gap from Crisis to Recovery

Understanding the Options for Therapy and Treatment

By Virgil Stucker

For many families we've worked with, their first encounter with mental illness was seeing odd behaviors or worrisome comments from a child or loved one, often developing slowly during adolescence. If these families were religious, their first attempt to get help may have been seeking advice from their priest, rabbi, minister, or imam or they may have turned to their general medical practitioner. They likely got referred to a local psychotherapist or psychiatrist in private practice. If the odd behaviors and worrisome comments continued, the family became more and more certain that their loved one had a mental illness. They would have sought a diagnosis, after which medication and/or psychotherapy may have been recommended.

Most times, the signs of mental illness seem to emerge out of the blue, most likely when the loved one is a young adult. The child who seemed to be excelling at school or work may suddenly not be. The symptoms of mental illness become extreme and even life-threatening. Perhaps there is abuse of legal or illegal substances. An emergency is declared. In the face of mental illness, families desperately seek understanding.

No matter which pattern applies to your family, it's likely that you're facing a situation where you are unsure what steps to take, what services are available, and what therapies might prove most effective.

To make matters worse, the private mental health care options often seem confusing and possibly unaffordable. The public mental health care options are often difficult to use because they are underfunded and understaffed. Medical insurance coverage focuses on "crisis stabilization." While improving due to recent court cases, payments for recovery-oriented care and treatment are still unpredictable.

As families and professionals team up to select where best to enter the continuum of care for a family member or patient, they assess things like diagnoses, level of acuity, complexity, willingness to participate and financial cost. In this chapter, we want to provide a big picture of the options you'll face. We'll start by talking about the journey itself so you'll understand what to expect. Then we'll go into more detail about the therapy options your loved one will have and the kinds of providers and treatment you may want to seek out depending on their situation and diagnoses. (We also note that you may actually be reading our words amidst the 8th, 9th or 10th crisis with your family member. You have not given up and you are still looking for hope.)

Understanding the Journey

The purpose of this book and of the work that we do is to help families and their loved one move out of the crisis stage in terms of mental health to the recovery stage. What does this mean?

- In the **crisis stage**, the person with the mental illness is living a life of chaos and confusion. They may be psychotic. They may have wild mood swings. They are unconnected to reality. There is a real concern that they pose a danger to themselves or to others. They are likely unable or unwilling to accept help when it is offered, unwilling or unable to participate in getting proper therapy and treatment.

- In the **recovery stage**, the person is not "cured." But they are living a life of meaning and purpose. They are connected with the world around them and have a sense of belonging. They are resilient, meaning they can bounce back if something throws them off track. With these factors working in their favor, they are able to sustain a high level of functioning and fulfillment.

Unfortunately, our current mental health systems do not make the transition from crisis to recovery easy. If the person's behaviors have not led to police intervention, someone in a crisis may be able to get short-term "crisis stabilization" support, if a bed is available. Whether voluntarily or involuntarily the young person is hospitalized in an inpatient acute care setting for this support. About a week later,[3] after the immediate danger has passed, the person is let go. Too often, their discharge plan is limited to a medication prescription and an appointment in a month with a local psychiatrist that they may never keep. A few hospitals may try to bridge the coming chasm of care with outpatient meetings for a few weeks, known as PHP or IOP, partial-hospital or intensive outpatient programs.

Once home, it's typical that the young person will end up playing video games all night and sleeping all day. They use their privacy protection to prevent their parents from getting any information about their diagnosis or treatments. They will

---

3   The average length of stay is 7.2 days per CDC.

usually stop taking any prescribed pills. Parents feel confused and concerned, expecting another crisis at any moment.

Without effective care, this pattern can continue for years. Rather than journeying toward recovery, a chronic state of illness may emerge. Reaching a point of sustained recovery seems impossible.

Once they discover that a quick cure is unlikely, the families of someone with a mental illness hope to map out a journey that avoids crises and helps to restore their family member's mental health. But as they look for answers, chaos and confusion may be nearly overwhelming.

What we want to make clear in this chapter is that the path from crisis to recovery is never as simple as we hope (see figure 1, top of next page). There will be progress and setbacks then progress again.

Figure 1: The Path from Crisis to Recovery

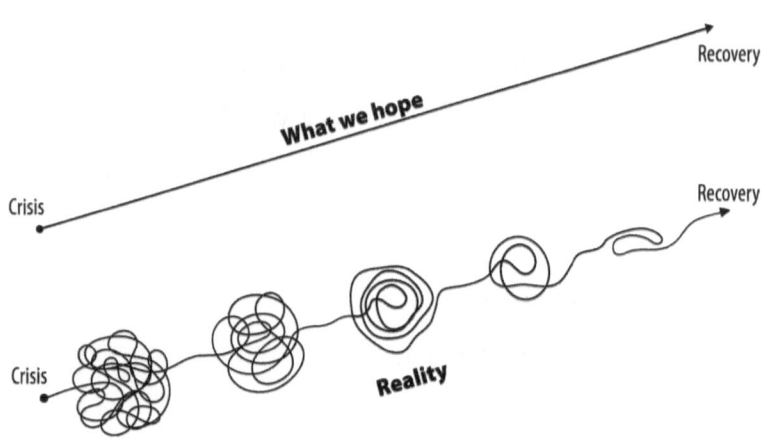

In the rest of this chapter, we want to help you sort through the confusion. We'll first talk about **therapy options**, meaning the *types* of treatments that may play a role in your loved one's recovery. Then we'll discuss what is often called the **continuum of care**, which means the range of services within which these therapies are available.

5 Therapy Options

There are five basic approaches used to reduce or control the symptoms of mental illness.

1. Psychological

Psychology-based therapies are most useful for people who like to think about and explore complex ideas about the mind and behavior.

These therapies most often involve meetings between the patient and a licensed psychologist or psychotherapist, where they talk about what's happening with the patient and develop strategies to control or counteract the effects of the illness. These meetings can be:

- Individual—just the patient and the therapist

- Group—several patients meet with the therapist at the same time

- Family—the patient and one or more family members meet with the family therapist.

There is also an option called **milieu therapy,** where the work between the patient and psychologists is done in the context of residential treatment (see p. 58 for more detail).

2. Medications (psychopharmacological or biochemical interventions)

Drugs and medications will generally play an important role in recovery for most people with a serious mental illness. The following kinds of biological treatments may be recommended to your loved one:

- Standard psychotropic medications for mental health symptoms ("psychotropic" means the medications affect the brain). This includes a wide range of drugs.

- The drug ketamine is sometimes mentioned as a potential therapy. It appears to help with depression in some patients but has no other confirmed effects.

- "Medically assisted treatment" (MAT)—these are medications given when the person is also getting counseling or behavior therapy for a persistent substance use disorder

- Using genetic information to better match medications with metabolism

There are other drug-related strategies that are currently being researched but are not ready for clinical use. These include the use of psychedelic drugs and more advanced gene therapy.

3. Neuroscientific or electromagnetic interventions

These therapies recognize that brain functions are electromagnetic as well as biochemical. There are three main types that are used for different kinds of mental illnesses. They are generally not the first options considered, but may be used if other treatments have been unsuccessful. See the table for their description. The "level of invasiveness" means how much the treatment intrudes into the body.

Level of invasive-ness	Therapy	Description	Primary uses
High	ECT (Electro-Convulsion Therapy)	Brief electrical stimulation is delivered to the brain while the patient is under anesthesia	Severe major depression Bipolar disorder that has not responded to other treatments
Medium	TMS trans-cranial magnetic stimulation	Uses magnetic fields to stimulate nerve cells in the brain	Depression that has resisted other treatments
Low	NFB Neuro-feedback (brain training)	Brain activity is monitored using sensors attached to the scalp	Attention disorders (ADD/ADHD) Post-traumatic stress disorder (PTSD)

4. Nutritional counseling for improved brain health

There is an increasing awareness of the impact that our diet has on our brain and mental functions.

- Five levels of nutritional psychiatry (See our Mental Horizons podcasts with Chris Palmer, MD and Georgia Ede, MD). Nutritional changes can improve brain and metabolic health of someone with a serious mental illness.

- The ketogenic diet—a specialized high-fat, low-carbohydrate diet, first devised decades ago to control epilepsy, is being prescribed by some psychiatrists to improve brain health. It is helping to diminish psychosis for some patients.

- Dietary supplements that may complement medications

5. Integrative Physical Health Interventions

As with diet, there is more and more evidence that physical health can impact mental health. This includes not just the level of physical activity but also the impact of injuries, disease, and pain on mental health. Options you may want to explore include:

- Developing an exercise routine for brain/body health

- Assessment and treatments of physical issues that may trigger mental health symptoms

- Assessment and treatment of pain

- Complementary treatments such as massage therapy, yoga, Qi Gong, and mindfulness training have been shown to be effective in diminishing symptoms of anxiety while enhancing general well-being.

Finding the Right Mix of Therapies

There are three lessons we want to pass on after reviewing the five major types of therapies that may play a role in your loved one's recovery:

- No single person should or could use all of therapy options we've just covered.

- There is no standard mix of therapies that will be good for everyone.

- There is no perfect recipe to address any specific diagnosis.

In short, the therapies you choose have to be matched to your loved one's situation, their symptoms, and their mental state and should be written into an overall recovery plan that indicates who is doing what by when to help your family member.

Involving your loved one in the discussion is critical because they must believe in the selected therapies. Not only will they be more likely to continue with therapies that they are convinced will help them, but their belief can create a placebo effect (improvement that happens even if the treatment is not the direct cause). It also helps if they are working with someone they trust—a pill offered by a prescriber who has a strong connection with your loved one will be more effective than one that comes from someone they don't know.

The Continuum of Care

Where (from whom) can you get these therapies? The answer is based on the complexity and acuity of the person's mental illness as assessed by a qualified clinician.

You will likely hear the term **continuum of care** when you deal with the mental health system. The term is defined in different ways depending on the situation. What all the definitions have in common is that they describe the range of services available to people dealing with mental health issues.

In this guide we're going to focus on a continuum that reflects the level of impact on the person with the mental illness and the person's mental state, as shown in Figure 2.

Figure 2: Continuum of Care

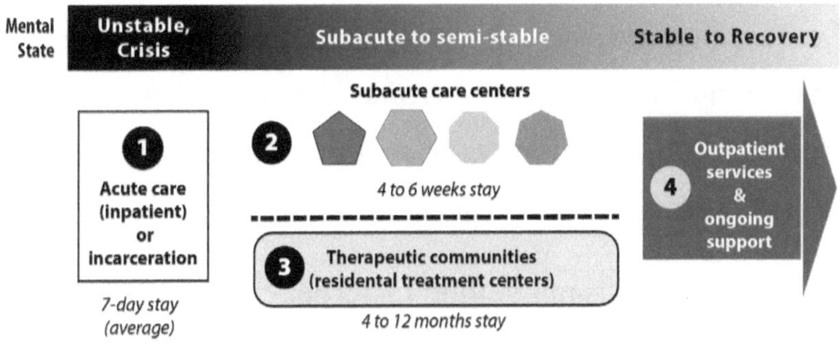

In the rest of this section, we'll go through each of the options following the numbered sequence.

1. Acute/Crisis Treatment

When someone is in crisis mode the only options are to put them in a facility capable of dealing with these extreme situations. In medical terms, their situation is labeled **acute**. As we discussed above, people in this state often cannot fully engage with the real world. They cannot evaluate their situation with logic and reason. They pose a danger to themselves or others, so they must be confined."

When someone is **acute and willing to accept care** they can gain access to inpatient care, generally in a local psychiatric hospital or in the psychiatric unit of a general hospital. (See the next page if your loved one is in a crisis but not willing to accept care.)

There are many private psychiatric hospitals; we tend to see better outcomes from those who are organized as nonprofits because they are more often oriented toward mission rather than money. The best choice is often the hospital that is closest to you, unless you have access to long-distance ambulance or secure transport services.

If your loved one is **not willing to accept care**, then involuntary care and/or incarceration may be indicated based on behavior. If the situation permits, contact an intervention professional for help. If not and you fear that danger is imminent, call 911—but note that **obtaining legal advice thereafter can be essential**. You may need to go through the court system to obtain what's called "emergency guardianship" so you can encourage the court to require involuntary care. This may give you more standing in the court if your family member is facing incarceration. Having guardianship also assures that your loved one cannot block you from being involved in their care and treatment. Hopefully, your family member will already have legal documents known as a **healthcare proxy** and **psychiatric advance directive** in place. If so, guardianship should not be needed. If not, make sure you help them create these documents as soon as they are able to more fully understand their situation.

2. Subacute inpatient care

People who are unstable and in distress but not considered to pose a danger to themselves or others are labeled as **subacute** by the medical system (or perhaps **semi-stable**). They "no longer meet the criteria," which means the system says that acute care in the mental health unit of a hospital is no longer "medically necessary." Once the "crisis has been stabilized," most medical insurance will no longer pay for continued inpatient care.

People in the subacute phase are often recovering from a crisis or they want to work on becoming more stable so they can avoid a crisis. (In reality, those who are recovering from a crisis were often discharged from inpatient hospitalization or incarceration before they were fully stable, perhaps to make room for other patients or inmates.)

For people in this situation, the best option may be **subacute treatment centers**, which are places where patients stay while receiving treatment focused on their conditions. The subacute stay generally lasts 4 to 6 weeks.

Subacute centers are residential, meaning the patients stay there 24/7 for some period of time. They provide intensive and often specialized services such as:

- **In-depth assessments**. Generally medications will have been increased during the hospital stay but in-depth assessments will not have been made. Fortunately, some of the "subacute" centers offer in-depth assessments.

- **Most or all of the therapies described earlier in this chapter.**

- **Programs for substance abuse.** These shorter-term, intensive treatments may be needed when the chaos created by substance abuse is more pronounced than the challenges posed by the person's mental illness. A "dual-diagnosis" (or co-occurring) program is best. One warning: "dual-diagnosis" programs should be carefully reviewed because they are often much better at treating substance abuse than mental health issues.

- **Niche treatments for trauma, personality disorders, eating disorders, and/or for obsessive-compulsive disorder.** Although these diagnoses are seldom isolated from accompanying diagnoses of mood disorders or psychosis, these short-term, niche programs may be useful when symptoms are extreme. Otherwise, it is generally better to utilize a more comprehensive program (see the discussion of residential communities later in this chapter).

Subacute care is expensive and not adequately covered by medical insurance, but may be helpful for unstable patients who do not meet the criteria for hospitalization in terms of posing a danger. This alternative provides a high level of safety, access to psychiatry and psychotherapy and adequate time for effective treatment, which used to be provided in longer-term hospital stays.

A danger for families is that their loved one ends up cycling through shorter-term, narrower, quick-fix options, going from one to the next, the next and the next... financially and emotionally exhausting themselves. To avoid this trap, do the best you can to make sure that the programs your loved one enters help them keep moving towards stable recovery.

3. Therapeutic communities (residential treatment)

People who are recovering from a crisis or who find subacute care insufficient have the option to go to a therapeutic community (also called residential treatment center). This option is most often used for people who have complex diagnoses or multiple illnesses (such as substance abuse along with mental illness).

People in those situations often benefit from longer-term treatment that combines many different disciplines. The treatment is focused both on teaching the individual how to cope successfully with their diagnosis while also defining and living out their dreams.

Residential treatment is sometimes described as a "recovery college," which is a good analogy. For one thing, the stay in a residential program may be longer than other forms of treatment, extending into 4 – 6 months or even a year or more. Longer stays provide opportunities to develop resiliency by putting new skills to the test in challenging, real-life but staff-supportive experiences. It also provides individuals both a respite from the overwhelming world and an opportunity to set their sights on improved functioning and fulfillment, while gaining a better sense of belonging, purpose and resiliency through skill development.

The best programs also provide "whole person" comprehensive care, rather than just narrowly focusing on symptoms, medications, etc. They often combine mental health science with a therapeutic/healing community milieu (drawn from the concept of "moral treatment, which we'll discuss in the next chapter).

Some of these therapeutic communities also offer professional support that approaches the subacute care options discussed above. The best centers also provide community re-integration services, often focused on returning to school and/or gaining employment, plus learning skills for independent living.

We note that families sometimes find these centers only after they have spent a great sum of money on quick fix options. They wish they had considered residential treatment sooner. For some families they should be a first choice, not a last chance. Residential treatment centers are also increasingly covered by medical insurance. Publicly funded group homes are also available; some are very good. Beware, however, of 'housing' that is more like warehousing.

4. Outpatient Services & Ongoing Support

Sometimes the person with mental illness does not need to receive residential treatment, through either subacute center or therapeutic communities. In other cases, they have made enough progress through the residential programs that they can move out and onward.

In both of these situations, the recovering person will be advised to continue a longer-term but less intensive relationship with an outpatient psychotherapist and/or a psychiatrist. Care managers can help to assure continued teamwork and arrange for needed outpatient support from local mental health professionals and often provide access to coaches. These professionals can help the recovering individual gain and stay in local employment or college, while perhaps transitioning from home to independent housing, often to a private apartment.

Once in the community, your family member may seek services from your local public mental health system which may also provide occasional access to a psychiatrist or a physician extender for prescriptions. (The potential danger here is that a lack of teamwork among providers can lead to the overuse of medication and inconsistent treatment objectives.)

Some of the most effective public mental health care is offered by ACT Teams (Assertive Community Treatment) also known as PACT (program of assertive community treatment). PACT brings together community-based treatment, rehabilitation, and support services to help stabilize people and allow even those with persistent mental illness to live independently. ACT/PACT programs sometimes work in alliance with Club Houses, which are designed to provide more chronically ill people with their highest quality of life. There are also some private PACT programs that provide enhanced support along with teams of coaches or mentors.

Dealing with the Unwilling Patient

Treatment options 2 through 4 that we just discussed are great if your loved is willing to accept help. But what if they aren't? This is a special, challenging category, especially if substance abuse is involved.

A good first step is often simply talking with your loved one. An open dialogue may help you discover what anxieties are preventing your loved one from seeking help. Listen deeply. Often we find that someone's statement that they don't need help is just a cover for their fears.

Other options you may want to explore are:

- **Tough love.** You may need to set and enforce specific boundaries, such as saying, "No, you can't live at home."

- Hiring a **mental health interventionist**, a highly trained and skilled professional who can sometimes persuade a greatly distressed person to accept the need for treatment.

- **Legal guardianship**, which may give you some temporary leverage but doesn't give you the right to force your family member to accept care and treatment against their will.

Support Services Needed on the Journey

Finding and getting the right kinds of therapies and treatments for your loved one is just part of the maze you have to navigate. At multiple points during the journey, you may also need to seek out the following kinds of services:

Comprehensive, therapeutic assessments. These assessments usually involve a thorough evaluation of an individual's physical, brain, and mental health along with the impact of any therapies they have received or are currently getting. If you want a comprehensive assessment, seek out experienced and credentialed practitioners. Some of the professionals work at residential (inpatient) settings, others provide outpatient evaluations, and some independent professionals travel to the family. The best professionals do not just assess the patient's status. They are also "therapeutic," which means that they help to engage the patient into accepting and participating in the recommended treatment options.

Legal navigation. Legal support is valuable at many points along the journey. Especially if your loved one is in a life-threatening crisis, you may need to obtain legal influence over their treatment decisions. That influence comes in three forms: guardianship, conservatorship, or trusteeship. Talk to your legal advisor to see which applies to your situation. You want to work with someone who can help you and your loved one complete helpful legal documents including a healthcare proxy, durable power of attorney, and an Advanced Psychiatric Directive. (Again, talk to your legal advisor to learn more about why these three documents are needed.) Legal advocacy can also help to open doors and to maximize access to medical insurance and to government-regulated benefits such as Medicaid and Social Security support.

Intervention and transport services. These services are sometimes literally the persuasive glue that holds the treatment and care processes together. They will help get your loved one to scheduled treatments, and can help you plan and carry out an intervention if needed. Some not only transport clients but also provide short-term, 24/7 supervised lodging in a hotel or AirBnB (for example, to house someone who would otherwise be at risk or relapsing or of slipping into a dangerous state of mind before they can be admitted for care.)

Long-term care planning for older clients. The ideal situation is to help individuals with complex psychiatric issues move into fully independent living, while achieving and sustaining their highest levels of functioning and fulfillment through some type of employment and life plan. But this is not always possible, especially for older adults or those with other conditions that make fully independent living risky. These people may need long-term care to continue their progress after they complete treatment at residential or subacute centers. There are only a few high-quality options for affordable long-term care. Additionally, some of the therapeutic or healing communities provide limited access to this option. Beware of custodial 'warehouses'; focus on options fostering continued, slower paced growth.

Long-term arrangements are most often accompanied by the formation of what's called a "discretionary trust," which can help to support a loved one's health and welfare beyond their parents' involvement. The trust should call for an annually reviewed recovery plan which may even provide financial incentives for your family member's continued goal achievements. While many different types of financial companies handle trusteeship and financial management of discretionary trusts, few seem willing to handle trusts where the beneficiary has a mental illness. Most professional or personal trustees may be encouraged to serve if the trust is designed to cover the cost for involving a mental health care coordinator in the decision making. When setting up the trust, you will also need an adept trust attorney who knows how to form the trust so that government benefits can be retained.

Public mental health care. The services offered by your state should not be forgotten. The public mental health system is all that most families in the US have access to either because of lack of finances or because of behaviors that prevent their inclusion in some of the programs listed above. The starting point may be your state's department of mental health website, which will show you the available services and how to enroll. In addition to the ACT programs listed above, you may learn about access to group homes and case managers. Resources for subsidized housing and support for seeking education and employment are available in some states. We have found some real 'stars' in the public system but acknowledge that most public systems are underfunded and understaffed.

Unfortunately, our jails and prisons are also a part of our public mental health system. Almost 400,000 people in our jails and prisons today have a psychiatric diagnosis and receive little if any care. Some of these inmates come from well-resourced families. Good attorneys and mental health advocates can sometimes help to get them into care options that may be accessible through mental health courts.

From Chaos to Calm

There are many roads to recovery, many paths from chaos to calm. The continuum presented here is not meant to capture all the potential options or provide specific answers for any particular individual or family. It is meant to give you a general overview of the options and possibilities.

As we've discussed before, there is no single answer for all. Even with a clear diagnosis, there is no one path, no perfect pill, no perfect, quick-fix program. The healing process takes time and often an integrative approach is required to meet the complex needs of each individual. The "pieces" need to be integrated into an overall recovery plan plotting out a continuous course of treatment and care.

This journey is never easy. For every success, there may be a setback. It helps to focus on the end goal of recovery (not cure!). Recovery embraces the hope and reality that people with complex diagnoses can achieve and sustain much higher levels of functioning and fulfillment. With the right plan and program, these individuals can have successful lives and achieve their dreams. Together with your family member and professionals you have to find the right formula to make that happen.

Chapter 4

An Uncertain Path:
Psychiatry from the 1700s to 1800s

By Stephanie McMahon

Chapters 4 and 5 may be a bit daunting for readers as they discover more of the imperfections in the history of mental health care. Many good people have been trying for centuries to help address and alleviate human distress and despair. These mental health scientists have labeled (diagnosed) the forms of mental illness in many different ways. Their treatment methods have ranged from caring and compassionate to gruesome, by today's standards. At times particular ideologies prevailed and some practitioners claimed they had perfect solutions. As the reader, you are already learning from us that perfect solutions do not exist. However, there are indeed individualized solutions that can lead to recovery. In reading chapters 4 and 5 you will see how the elements of these solutions have been emerging over time. As a resilient champion and caregiver, your knowledge of the imperfect history, as well as new, emerging solutions, will help you advise and support your loved one as he or she weaves together the elements of their best plan for recovery in conjunction with advice from the mental health professionals who are on their team.

For as long as humans have existed, mental illness has existed. What's changed over time is how we have labeled and responded to mental illness. Society has sometimes reacted with horror; sometimes with awe. Sometimes we have embraced the mentally ill; more often rejected them.

To fully understand why the mental health system today functions the way it does, it helps to understand the history. We'll go back about 250 years from today to shed light on the question, "How did we end up where we are now?" Hindsight reveals methods in the past that today may seem barbaric. Back then, they were the best that the compassionate minds of the time could devise. "Where we are now" is still far from perfect and we still strive to improve.

- This chapter reviews the beginnings of psychiatry as a field of medicine. This was also a time when people began to think of mental illness as something to be viewed with compassion instead of fear.

- The next chapter will dive into the more recent history of psychiatry covering from about 1900 to today.

Mental Illness During the 18th Century: The great confinement

Let's travel back to the late 1700s. In Western civilization it is a time when the faith and superstition of the Middle Ages are being replaced by belief in reason and logic. That's why it's called the Age of Reason or the Age of Enlightenment. It was also around this time that the human population on Earth surpassed one billion people for the first time and densely populated cities were a new norm.

In the Middle Ages, people believed that those suffering from a mental illness were possessed by demons. During the Enlightenment, people began to wonder if there was a scientific reason behind mental illness. Then, as now, society understood that there was a spectrum of severity from mild to extreme. To find those with the more extreme cases, you would look in four main places:

- The private homes of families wealthy enough to care for someone in this state

- The churches charged with the care of these individuals

- The homeless poor living marginal lives on the streets

- The locked rooms in hospitals where these individuals were confined

As you can see, there was no central or organized approach (or understanding) to the treatment of mental illness at that time. The often well-meaning but harmful actions of families, churches, and hospitals meant that the mentally ill were separated from society, destined to live in isolation. Living apart meant their ability to work or connect meaningfully with others was greatly limited. If there is one thing we know that is essential to all human health, it is social connection. In addition, the fact that the mentally ill were hidden away led to some horrible abuses.

Fortunately, all of that was about to change in ways that still affect our approach to mental illness today.

Moral Treatment & Asylums: A more ethical approach

At the end of the 1700s, a physician in France named Philippe Pinel and a Quaker in England named William Tuke became champions for more humane and ethical care of the mentally ill. Their ideas were a radical departure from the brutality and confinement of the 1600s and early to mid-1700s.

Pinel used the term **moral treatment** to describe this philosophy. It was a paternalistic model where the mentally ill were treated very much like children who had to be taken care of. Pinel believed that insane people did not need to be chained or beaten, but instead treated with kindness, offered freedoms, and allowed access to recreation, conversation, and light manual labor.

The Growth of Asylums

Moral treatment emphasized the importance of the environment as being the main therapeutic tool to help people relearn how to be participants in everyday life. The desire to create a better environment for the mentally ill led to the creation of the first asylums in the late 1700s.

The original impulse behind the asylum was to create a place of secure refuge. In fact, that is the root definition of the word asylum and the driving force behind the moral treatment movement. Much like an immigrant fleeing their country, the person experiencing psychosis is unmoored from their life and in need of a secure refuge, a place of rest and sanctuary.

Asylums were viewed as places where people could go when their mental condition kept them from being able to live on their own. An asylum was somewhere a person could get protection, rest, and care.

Moral treatment included a rigid daily schedule, having patients and staff dining together and access to creative outlets such as arts and crafts. Moral treatment also valued the therapeutic use of labor, which is why many asylums included woodshops, gardens, farms, and orchards with work assignments based on gender.

The asylum as a specialized institution for the containment of the mentally ill became increasingly popular in Western society during the 1800s. Initially, asylums were mostly run by churches; later by physicians or medical specialists of that time known as superintendents of the asylum.

While moral treatment led to more humane treatment, the explosive growth of asylums reflected the Age of Reason belief that the mentally ill needed to be separated from the rest of society. This led French philosopher Michel Foucault to coin the term "The Great Confinement" to describe this period in history.

The first proponent of moral treatment in the U.S. was Benjamin Rush, a physician and humanitarian. He believed that the insane should be treated in a bucolic hospital setting away from the busy pace of everyday life. Rush also employed medical practices such as blood-letting and he invented the "tranquilizer chair" as a restraint.

In the mid-1800s, after Rush's death, Dorothea Dix continued the push for hospitals to be spacious, with lots of light and beautiful grounds. Because of her activism and efforts, there was much optimism in the 1840s and 1850s. It was believed that allowing people with mental illness to live without restraints in a peaceful setting and having a highly structured schedule would help cure their disease.

The Beginning of the End of Asylums

While "cures" did not happen, the popularity of asylums and mental hospitals continued to grow. By the second half of the 1800s, there was a lot of pressure on mental hospitals to admit more and more patients. While initially only the mentally ill were confined in asylums, eventually prostitutes, blasphemers, vagrants, and others deemed "undesirable" were also locked away against their will.

The growth in the number of people confined in mental hospitals began to strain the system. The original vision of moral treatment was of small facilities of no more than 30 patients, with stays most often being of a year or less. These were initially framed as meaningful, healing experiences with superintendents researching outcomes and showing improvements. This original vision fell away as asylums turned into large facilities housing thousands of patients for years at a time (and often lifetimes). With that many people, little attention was given to patients as individuals and it became impossible to properly maintain buildings and grounds.

With this shift, one could no longer call these large state hospitals "asylums". The early efforts to create effective, compassionate therapeutic communities ended. During this period of overcrowding, interest in "curing" mental illness came to the forefront. As a result, these expanding state mental hospitals became the location for decades of medical experiments to find cures, conducted on largely unwilling and uninformed individuals.

And yet, the persistent problem of overcrowding and poor treatment of patients was leading the public to question whether these large state institutions were the best way to provide care for people with severe mental illness.

Psychiatry as a New Field of Academic Study

In the mid-1800s, the German scientist Wilhelm Griesinger created the first ties between an asylum and a university clinic. Before Griesinger, psychiatry was a small component of the academic medical world. Griesinger was instrumental in launching the field of psychiatry as a respected discipline worthy of academic study.

Griesinger was a strong proponent of the new perspective that mental illness was a disorder of the brain and nerves. As this belief took hold, research into brain anatomy moved to the fore. Researchers like Alois Alzheimer discovered abnormalities in the brain, such as plaques and tangles.

In this same era, another German researcher, Emil Kraepelin, observed people living in the asylums. As a result of his research, he devised a classification system for mental illness that divided it into two main categories:

- Dementia praecox (later labeled schizophrenia)

- A catch-all category of manic-depressive psychosis

Kraepelin's[4] work was the first time that mental illness was seen not as a simple continuum of one illness, but rather as a collection of different diseases.

The basic scientific work of Griesinger and Alzheimer made no contribution to actual clinical care for people. On the contrary, this new model of German psychiatry was pessimistic and saw mental illness as a chronic state of decline. Kraepelin's research was consistent with this view, leading to the widespread belief that there was no hope of change for people suffering from a mental illness.

---

4   In later years, Kraepelin was criticized for his belief in eugenics, as practice that played a key role in Nazi philosophy.

The Turn of the 20th Century: Freud vs. the anatomists

It wasn't until the work of Sigmund Freud, between 1895 and 1905, that the idea of making symbolic meaning of mental illness returned to the public discourse.

Freud was a **psychoanalyst**, someone who believes that mental illness is the result of events in our lives, not just our biology. He believed that exploring the unconscious mind by talking and listening (psychoanalysis) could lead the distressed person to gain insights about the causes of their mental illness and develop strategies to address them.

These views were in sharp contrast to the **anatomists** (like the German researchers we just discussed) who thought there were physical explanations for mental illness. This idea was supported when many soldiers returning from World War I were unable to cope with civilian life. Their condition was called shell-shock at the time (later called PTSD). The idea that explosions had caused shell shock by rattling the brain added support to the concept that mental illness had a biological root cause. Anatomists had little use for the symbolism of psychoanalysis and Freud's work of finding meaningful psychological causes for mental illness.

Despite these criticisms, Freud's work has had a massive impact on Western culture, affecting everything from literature and advertising to cinema and child-rearing. Especially after his death in 1939, his general ideas were extended to treatments for all types of mental illness, mild to severe.

However, in the United States, scorn for Freud's views continued to grow in the early 1900s among those in the psychiatric field and his theories were not widely adopted. A tension between these two perspectives was maintained for decades, with the anatomists and the psychoanalysts vying for dominance.

Experimenting on the Mentally Ill

One of the downsides of the anatomical view of mental illness was that it led to widespread experimentation on how to physically alter the brain. The ideas most widely tested at first were that mental illness could be shocked or cut out of the body somehow.

These ideas came to fore in the first half of the 1900s in America when "...therapeutic experimentation on the vulnerable bodies of those certified mad..." was methodically carried out (Andrew Scull, *Madness: A very short introduction*, 2011).

At this time, state mental hospitals still housed the most severely ill, who had few rights and no ability to refuse treatment or experimentation. The list of testing done on these people in hopes of finding a physical cure to mental illness is frightening. It included experiments using drugs, electricity, malarial mosquitoes to induce fever, partial drowning, spinning chairs, insulin coma, 5-point restraints, sensory deprivation, the surgeon's scalpel, and noxious gas.

The Lobotomy

Perhaps the worst of all the treatments investigated in this era was a method invented in the 1930s by a Portuguese scientist, Antonio Moniz. He developed a procedure called a **prefrontal lobotomy**. He would first bore a hole in the skull of a patient with a mental illness, then use a tool that looked very much like a butter knife to make cuts in the prefrontal cortex of the brain.

Two medical school doctors, Walter Freeman and James Watts, studied with Moniz and brought the prefrontal lobotomy to the US. Their method involved boring into the brain through the eye socket with an ice-pick-like device and a mallet to damage the brain.

Though these procedures sound (and were) horrible, lobotomies quickly became popular because they did usually get rid of psychosis. Society at that time did not seem too concerned that people who had lobotomies also lost the capacity for empathy, forethought, and impulse-control. In addition, their personalities were often irreversibly altered. The procedure was done on patients as young as 4 years old and was carried out regularly at US hospitals.

Setting the Stage for the Modern Era

By the early 1900s, psychiatry was being pulled in different directions.

- Massive state mental hospitals were still used to house large numbers of people with severe forms of mental illness, but there was increasing discomfort with this model of care.

- The psychiatrists and psychoanalysts were presenting opposing views of the causes and cures for mental illness.

- Most researchers in the field were exploring brain function, but this led to inhumane experimentation on unwilling patients.

These forces set the stage for rapid changes in psychiatry during the middle to late 20th century, which we will discuss in the next chapter.

Chapter 5

Struggles & Hope:
Psychiatry in the Modern Era

By Stephanie McMahon

Throughout the latter part of the 20th century, the desire to achieve moral treatment for people with mental illness began to reshape the discipline. There were many advances and many setbacks that led to three trends:

- The search for chemical cures (increasing use of drugs)

- The demise of large state hospitals

- The move away from psychoanalysis to psychiatry

In this chapter, we'll discuss each of these trends, then talk about the imperfect but improved solutions that have taken the place of older treatments.

Trend 1: Drug therapies and the search for a magical chemical bullet

In 1928, penicillin was discovered. The excitement of the discovery of a drug-based therapy to treat infections bled into other areas of science, including psychiatry.

The public had begun to understand that mental illness was a product of imbalanced brain chemistry, neurotransmitters misfiring, and bad genes. Then in the late 1940s, a tiny French drug company called Rhone-Poulenc began experimenting with a drug called chlorpromazine. Use of the drug was soon referred to as a "chemical lobotomy" because it had the same effect as a prefrontal lobotomy when given to people with severe psychosis. That is, the psychosis disappeared (along with the other effects described in the previous chapter.)

The drug rights for chlorpromazine were sold to an American company called Smith, Kline, and French, who renamed the drug Thorazine. It eventually became the first antipsychotic drug.

Thorazine was no penicillin, but it ushered in a new era of psychiatry that included a stunning rate of medication development for every type of mental ailment. As of 1953, Thorazine had been tested on a grand total of 104 psychiatric patients, without their consent. Thirteen months later, thanks to the subduing effects of the drug, it was being prescribed to over 2 million people.

The pharmaceutical industry exploded in growth from this point forward. Many other drugs used to treat psychosis were soon developed. The pharmaceutical industry then popularized tranquilizers, the next big wave of medications for curing mental ills. By the mid-1970s, Valium, part of a new class of medications called benzodiazepines, was the most prescribed (and abused) medication in many countries (benzodiazepines are sedatives and tranquilizers).

In that time period, the understanding of mental illness continued to expand. For example, "anxiety" was a very popular diagnosis. Slowly, psychiatrists began to use the label of "depression" as the most popular diagnosis. Antidepressants such as Prozac rose in popularity and use. Both anxiety and depression encompassed definitions of mental stress, tension, and discomfort that gave rise to a more generalized experience of mental illness, with much of the general public sometimes meeting criteria for a mental illness that did not exist a few years earlier.

Today, the medication class of opioids is in the spotlight, much like Valium and other benzodiazepines were in the 1970s. In contrast to Valium-like drugs, opioids are used for the relief of pain. More than a third of drug overdoses today involve a combination of benzodiazepines and opioids.

It is important to note that the pharmaceutical industry is the single most profitable industry in the world. In 2008, antipsychotics alone accounted for $14.6 billion dollars in annual profit.

The Full Cost of the Drugs

Now in 2020, our understanding of the brain is still in its infancy. We continue to know very little about the causes of psychosis, schizophrenia, or bipolar disorder. We are also still struggling to find optimal medication regimens, which means finding the *least* amount of the right kinds of drugs to achieve the desired effects. In order to select the most effective medications, it is more and more important also to take time to develop a deeper understanding through comprehensive assessments, which can include a genetic analysis which helps to match medications with one's metabolism.

While this approach sounds good in principle, there is an overlooked cost to individuals and to society: an epidemic in the problems that these drugs can create for people with mental illness if they are over-medicated and are not counseled in ways to avoid some of the side effects. Many of the drugs are well known to correlate with heart disease, metabolic dysfunction, brain damage, weight gain, and diabetes, to name just a few. People with serious mental illness who use these drugs may have a lower life expectancy by 15 to 25 years, on average, compared to the general population. There may be other factors contributing to this shortened lifespan, such as the effects of the mental illness itself, suicide, physical inactivity and poor nutrition. But the medications are also implicated. This is the most jagged pill to swallow.

Trend 2: The shift towards psychiatry and away from psychoanalysis

Before the 1950s, the majority of psychiatrists worked in mental hospitals. As large state hospitals lost favor and began to shut down, droves of psychiatrists left to work in outpatient settings and private practice, where they could work with relatively stable people.

As the emphasis shifted more and more to the use of drugs, the pharmaceutical industry started paying academic institutions to conduct experiments with new medications.

A new thought also emerged that combined the practice of psychoanalysis and psychotherapy with the use of antipsychotics and other medications: if you can control the symptoms of mental illness with drugs, a person may be more able and willing to pursue the underlying causes of their illness through talk therapy.

However, as pharmaceutical funding for research increased, the field of psychiatry soon started getting much more attention than psychoanalysis and psychotherapy. In colleges and universities, the position of department head that used to be filled by psychoanalysts was rapidly replaced with psychiatrists working as neuroscientists and psychopharmacologists.

Psychiatry brought with it a more systematized approach to mental illness, which largely alienated psychoanalysts. Building on Kraepelin's work, which identified two broad categories of mental illness, by 1952, the first Diagnostic and Statistical Manual (DSM) was published. It detailed a total of 106 unique mental health diagnoses. This expansion continued throughout the latter half of the 20th century:

- DSM-I in 1952: 106 diagnostic categories

- DSM-II in 1968: 182 categories

- DSM-III in 1980: 265 categories

- DSM-IV in 1994: 297 categories

There is a cynical explanation for this rapid increase in the number of diagnostic categories. As Scull wrote, "The more precise the diagnostic criteria, the more easily pharmaceutical companies could create and market medications for specific psychiatric use." (More recently, the psychiatric profession received heavy criticism about the constantly growing number of diagnostic categories. The most recent revision, the DSM-5, was published in 2013 and also includes 297 diagnostic categories.)

Interestingly, when the DSM-III was published in 1980, it made almost no mention of Freudian or psychoanalytic terms. The goal of psychiatry shifted to detecting scientific markers and symptoms of the different diseases.

The 1990s was declared The Decade of the Brain by the National Institute of Mental Health (NIMH). The fall of psycho-analysis as the dominant philosophy in psychiatry made way in the latter half of the 20th century for a mix of biological, social, and psychological approaches to treatment.

Trend 3: Out of the large state hospitals and onto the streets (or into prisons)

In 1955, the number of patients in state psychiatric hospitals in the U.S. peaked at 559,000.

The arrival of Thorazine coincided with great public criticism of the state of these large institutions post-WWII. This led to a change in public policy and thousands of patients were discharged within a short period of time. Over the years that followed, most state hospitals closed permanently as funding dried up and interest turned to community-based care. (Some beds often remained available for the most dangerous fo-rensic patients.)

At the same time that these large institutions fell out of favor in the US, the same was happening in other countries, including England, France, and Spain.

When hundreds of thousands of psychiatric patients were discharged from these crumbling structures, one of three things happened to them:

- The new medications allowed some to manage their symptoms independently and lead stable lives.

- Other patients found the combination of outpatient care and medications to be adequate enough to help them live relatively stable lives. Many of these individuals returned to living with family members.

- Patients with more severe or chronic issues and who had no family were suddenly homeless. They were exposed to the trials of the street: illicit drugs, starvation, incarceration, violence, and premature death.

Prisons: The new confinement

For those enduring the most severe and persistent mental illness, the negative toll from the loss of large public institutions was extreme. The US courts and government leaders, after essentially closing the brick-and-mortar hospitals, failed to provide the promised funding to establish community care centers in each state,as had been envisioned by President Kennedy.

To this day, no state in the US provides the minimum number of recommended inpatient psychiatric beds to meet the needs of its citizens. And no state has been successful in establishing an adequate number of community mental health centers to meet the demand for outpatient therapy.

A report written by the Treatment Advocacy Center in 2018 stated that,

> *"The United States is effectively running 50 different experiments, with no two states taking the same approach. As a result, whether or not an individual receives timely, appropriate treatment for an acute psychiatric crisis or chronic psychiatric disease is almost entirely dependent on what state he or she is in when the crisis arises."*

A new kind of confinement has occurred: prisons, which house about 400,000 mentally ill inmates. Today in California, prisons are the largest "providers" of mental health care. Thankfully, many states have diversion programs established to interrupt the now well-worn path of psychiatric patients from the Emergency Room to a jail cell.

Today's Options

Today, public state mental hospitals are nearly extinct and specialized residential treatment programs only partially fill the role that had been envisioned for the first asylums. State mental hospitals all over the country are shuttered. And as we discussed earlier, no state in the US provides enough inpatient psychiatric beds to meet demand. It is no wonder why families feel they are not getting enough support.

We have developed an impressive array of medication and therapeutic treatments for mental illness, but a cure still eludes us. A lot of important strides have been made in our understanding of the brain, including the connection between the brain and the gut microbiome, but more studies are needed and funds are scarce.

The field of **integrative psychiatry**—which sees the symptoms of mental illness as signs that systems in the body are out of balance—is gaining in popularity. In many ways, we have made progress in small pockets of the field and have evolved our understanding of mental illness in small but significant ways.

From the acute and subacute treatment centers to outpatient services and residential communities discussed in Chapter 3, treatment is more patient-centered now than ever. These small ways need a bigger spotlight in order to grow and take root if they are to contend with the population disease burden of mental illness currently weighing on almost every country around the world.

Pockets of Hope

When you look at the evolution of psychiatry from a 40,000-foot vantage, it is easy to miss all the good that has happened. In the midst of today's patchwork of solutions, small pockets of hope exist where people are given respect, shown kindness, and cared for in holistic ways.

Where are those places, who are those champions, and how can we draw public attention to their efforts? They are not flashy, quick-fixes or miracle cures. We've learned our lesson with those kinds of things, right?

The last fifteen years or so have seen a new generation of antipsychotic drugs, with better therapeutic effects and fewer side effects. But there is still too much emphasis on chemical treatment of diseases like schizophrenia.

A decade ago, the late Oliver Sacks, MD wrote for the "New York Review of Books" about some pockets of hope in the mental health field. You can hear the echo of Pinel's and Tuke's philosophy in Sacks' words:

> *"What is the situation now? The state hospitals that still exist are almost empty and contain only a tiny fraction of the numbers they once had. The remaining inmates consist for the most part of chronically ill patients who do not respond to medication or incorrigibly violent patients who cannot be safely allowed outside. The vast majority of mentally ill people, therefore, live outside mental hospitals. Some live*

alone or with their families and visit outpatient clinics, and some stay in "halfway houses," residencies that provide a room, one or more meals, and the medications that have been prescribed.

Such residences vary greatly in quality—but even in the best of them (as brought out by Tim Parks in his review of Jay Neugeboren's book about his schizophrenic brother, Imagining Robert, and by Neugeboren himself, in his recent review of The Center Cannot Hold, Elyn Saks's autobiographical account of her own schizophrenia), patients may feel isolated and, worst of all, scarcely able to get the psychiatric advice and counseling they may need.

The last fifteen years or so have seen a new generation of antipsychotic drugs, with better therapeutic effects and fewer side effects, but the too exclusive an emphasis on "chemical" models of schizophrenia, and on purely pharmacological approaches to treatment, may leave the central human and social experience of being mentally ill untouched.

Particularly important in New York City—especially since deinstitutionalization—is Fountain House, which was established sixty years ago, and provides a clubhouse on West 47th Street for mentally ill people from all over the city.

Here they can come and go freely, meet others, eat communally, and, most importantly, be helped to secure jobs and fill out tax forms and tricky paperwork of one sort or another.

Similar clubhouses have now been established in many cities. There are dedicated staff members and volunteers at these *clubhouses, but they are crucially dependent on private funds, and these have been less forthcoming during the current recession.*

There are also, intriguingly, certain residential communities that derive, historically, both from the asylums and the therapeutic farm communities of the nineteenth century, and these provide, for the fortunate few who can go to them, comprehensive programs for the mentally ill. I have visited some of these—Gould Farm in Massachusetts, CooperRiis in North Carolina—and seen in them much of what was admirable in the life of the old state hospitals: community, companionship, opportunities for work and creativity, and respect for the individuality of everyone there, now coupled with the best of and whatever medication is needed.

Often it is rather modest medication in these ideal circumstances. Many of the patients in such places (though they may remain schizophrenic or bipolar for the rest of their lives, in the sense that a diabetic remains a diabetic) may graduate after several months or perhaps a year or two, and be able to lead full and satisfying lives with no relapses, no recidivism, no looking back.

But there are only a handful of comparable facilities in the US—they can accommodate no more than a few hundred patients out of the millions that exist. These patients must depend on their families to help pay the very considerable costs of staying there—more than $100,000 a year—and on whatever can be raised from private sources.

The remainder—the 99 percent of the mentally ill who have insufficient resources of their own—must face inadequate treatment and lives that cannot reach their potential. The National Alliance for the Mentally Ill does what it can, but the millions of mentally ill remain the least supported, the most disenfranchised, and the most excluded people in our society today.

And yet it is clear—from the experiences of places like CooperRiis and Gould Farm, and of individuals like Elyn Saks—that schizophrenia is not necessarily a relentlessly deteriorating illness (although it can be); and that, in ideal circumstances, and when resources are available, even the most deeply ill people—who have been relegated to a "hopeless" prognosis—may be enabled to live satisfying and productive lives."

Other Resources

Fountain House, CooperRiis, and Gould Farm all made Oliver Sacks' list of best programs in the U.S. We would add Spring Lake Ranch in Vermont, Hopewell Community in Ohio, Rose Hill Center in Michigan and Windhorse, founded in Colorado and now with locations in Massachusetts, Oregon, California, Germany, Austria, and Italy.

We would also include the 30+ member programs of the American Residential Treatment Association (ARTA). Many are non-profit organizations that rely not only on fees but on significant donations to keep their doors open and their programs running.

Another program that has much promise for scalability and wrap-around community care for those most persistently ill is the Program of Assertive Community Treatment (PACT) model such as what McLean Hospital opened in 2018.

These are the pockets of hope, the places where kindness and compassion are just as important as treatment plans and medication usage.

The Increasing Burden on Families

Look back 200 years, to the time right before asylums gained wide popularity, and you'd see today what you saw then: most people with mental illness are living in the homes of families or are out on the streets.

What progress can we say has actually been made? When asylums disappeared, very little took their place. The burden of care was tossed like a hot potato from the federal to the state to the local level and finally, the family.

The kinds of treatment centers discussed above are ideal, but these options are not available to families who can not afford them, who do not have medical insurance to pay for them, or who are not fortunate enough to have their family member accepted at one that offers scholarships. The question of how to pay for these comprehensive programs is very real. The large mental hospitals were, for the most part, federally funded. When they closed, the financial burden of care passed to the state and then the local level.

Today, if you have an adult child with a serious mental illness, you have to accept whatever public assistance is available in your state. Or you have to take on the financial burden yourself of paying for a private program. And/or you become politically active, pushing for reforms, or you become philanthropically active, bonding with other families to create your own program.

Families are also organizing to force medical insurance companies to be more helpful. Insurance companies have been very slow to cover residential treatment despite the Mental Health Parity and Addiction Equity Act of 2008, which required insurers and providers to approach mental health benefits the same way they approach medical or surgical benefits. Some recent class action court cases are beginning to force insurance companies to be faster in responding to their duty and to the law. Headway is being made, although it is an uphill struggle for parity-seekers. Organizations like the Treatment Advocacy Center are helping to hold the feet of insurance companies to the fire and advance policies and practices around mental health parity.

Are We Meeting the Moral Test of a Society?

This guide is written for the families who may be beginning the journey or who may, for years, have been caring for a loved one with serious mental illness. It honors all the individuals whose rights to a fulfilling life were stolen away by extreme interventions forced on them against their will.

Once you listen to enough individual stories and listen to the news, it's not a leap to conclude that our mental health system in the U.S. is in crisis. This is especially true when it comes to people whose needs require coordination between many specialists, disciplines, and healthcare systems. As a result, it can be difficult for people with worsening mental health concerns to receive the support they need in a timely manner.

Parents and supporters of people with behavioral health problems, substance abuse, or mental health issues want to have easy access to credible, trustworthy, and unbiased resources for support. They need help in determining what is appropriate for their child or family member and how they may access the best services to fit their needs.

Hubert Humphrey, US Vice President from 1965 to 1969, spoke about the treatment of the weakest members of society as a reflection of its government:

"...the moral test of government is how that government treats those who are in the dawn of life, the children; those who are in the twilight of life, the elderly; those who are in the shadows of life; the sick, the needy and the handicapped."

When we closed the large mental institutions, we removed a critical load-bearing structure in our society that accepted the burden of care. Now that burden rests on families. And more often than not, it breaks families apart, pushing people to their very limits, draining financial and emotional resources. We need to do better. In our pursuit of proving the cause and finding a cure for mental illness, we have severely neglected the very individuals we sought to help in the first place.

The Next Step

The next step forward includes you at the front: individuals experiencing mental illness and families who support these individuals. The family unit is the heart of our society and the place where we learn about the value of human connection. We do not believe there is a cure for mental illness, but we know for certain that mental illness thrives on isolation.

The antidote to isolation is connection. The path forward must include a broader awareness in society about the importance of real connections, respect for meeting individual needs for those in recovery, and an acceptance of the spectrum of human experience. We are a diverse rainbow of humans and a diverse array of recovery options delivered in person-centered environments is the future of mental health treatment.

About the Authors

Virgil Stucker. Virgil is a visionary, mission-focused, non-profit leader with over 30 years of experience focused on the healing power of community, creativity, and philanthropy. He has served as Executive Director and/or President of seven not-for-profit organizations and founding board member of several others. He was also a turn-around agent for a health care system, a professor for master's students in philanthropy, and is a consultant to other visionaries. Virgil is the founder and president of Virgil Stucker and Associates LLC, a therapeutic consulting practice that empowers clients in their mental health decision making. Virgil splits his time between Massachusetts and North Carolina with his wife, Lis. They are the proud parents of four grown children and seven grandchildren (with the 8th to arrive in April 2020). Virgil plays the saxophone and Native American flute in his free time. Virgil graduated Phi Beta Kappa in philosophy from Ripon College and holds an MBA in nonprofit leadership and management for Western New England University.

Stephanie McMahon, MA. Stephanie is a health communications specialist and a certified health coach. She has been working in the mental health and nonprofit fields for over 15 years. She holds a Master's degree in communications from Johns Hopkins University where her studies focused on health literacy. She is a graduate of the Functional Medicine Coaching Academy. Stephanie is a lifelong learner, always researching the latest in integrative health approaches to diet, stress management, sleep, and ancestral health practices. Above all else, Stephanie believes in the power of social connection as the matrix from which healing begins. She resides on a farm in Western Massachusetts with her husband and two teenage children and enjoys hiking, foraging, and cooking.

References

Foucalt, Michel. *Madness and Civilization: a History of Insanity in the Age of Reason*. Vintage Books, 1961.

Sacks, Oliver. "The Lost Virtues of the Asylum." *The New York Review of Books*, 2009, www.nybooks.com/articles/2009/09/24/the-lost-virtues-of-the-asylum/.

Scull, Andrew. *Madness: a Very Short Introduction*. Oxford University Press, 2011.

www.ingramcontent.com/pod-product-compliance
Lightning Source LLC
Chambersburg PA
CBHW021440210526
45463CB00002B/592